BE HEALTH WITH REFLEXOLOGY

Enjoy an Alternative Medicine to Improve your Health!

ZSUZSANNA T. GROUNDS

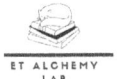

ET ALCHEMY
LAB

CONTENTS

Introduction	vii
1. CHAPTER 1. Introduction To Reflexology	1
2. CHAPTER 3. Benefits	14
3. CHAPTER 4. Extreme Emotions: The Effects	20
4. CHAPTER 5. The Reflexology Chart Map	24
5. CHAPTER 6. How To Practice Reflexology	34
6. Chapter 7. The Whole-Body Reflexology	41
7. CHAPTER 8. Reflexology Techniques	48
8. Conclusions	53

© **Copyright 2021 – Zsuzsanna T. Grounds- All rights reserved.**

The content contained within this book may not be reproduced, duplicated or transmitted without direct written permission from the author or the publisher.

Under no circumstances will any blame or legal responsibility be held against the publisher, or author, for any damages, reparation, or monetary loss due to the information contained within this book. Either directly or indirectly.

Legal Notice:

This book is copyright protected. This book is only for personal use. You cannot amend, distribute, sell, use, quote or paraphrase any part, or the content within this book, without the consent of the author or publisher.

Disclaimer Notice:

Please note the information contained within this document is for educational and entertainment purposes only. All effort has been executed to present accurate, up to date, and reliable, complete information. No warranties of any kind are declared or implied. Readers acknowledge that the author is not engaging in the rendering of legal, financial, medical or professional advice. The content within this book has been derived from various sources. Please consult a licensed professional before attempting any techniques outlined in this book.

By reading this document, the reader agrees that under no circumstances is the author responsible for any losses, direct or indirect, which are incurred as a result of the use of information contained within this document, including, but not limited to, — errors, omissions, or inaccuracies.

INTRODUCTION

You might feel powerless in your existence today, especially when you are dealing with your usual daily stresses. When your body is disordered, you might run to grab the nearest pill and put it in your mouth. It is not necessary to do this yet. One way to deal with your daily routine is reflexology, which is an alternative medicine that involves applying pressure to your hands, feet, or ears using finger, hand, and thumb-specific techniques that may or may not contain lotion or oil.

Reflexology is based on a system of reflective zones and zones that reflect the image of the human body on your hands and feet, with the premise that a reflexology session can affect a positive physical change on your body. While reflexology does not replace conventional medicine, it can help you manage your symptoms. It can help yourself to reduce stress.

This book talks about the basics of reflexology and its advantages for you. It also documents the long history of the method and how different forms have emerged. When you're done reading this book, you'll gain a new understanding of what reflexology is. It is not just a relaxing massage. It's also a way to reduce your anxiety and stress. If you suffer from a disease, a reflexology session can help you a great deal.

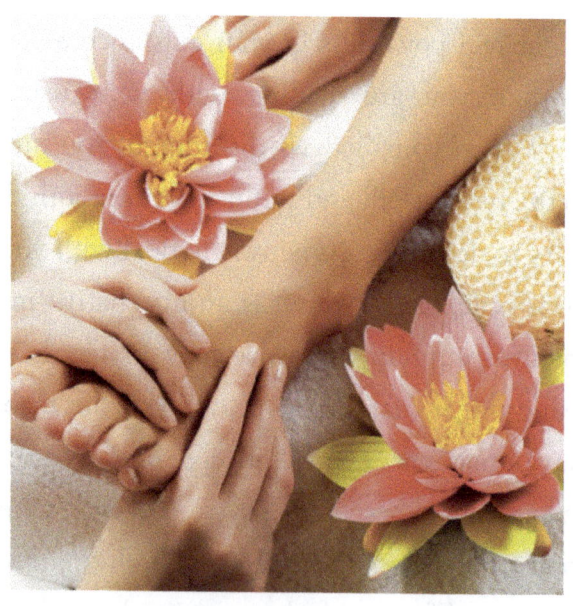

CHAPTER 1. INTRODUCTION TO REFLEXOLOGY

Reflexology is a form of healing that aims to improve an individual's overall health. It is non-invasive and easy to practice. Most professional reflexologists were simply patients who had felt the effectiveness of the method. After several sessions with a reflexologist, most people decide to learn why reflexology is so effective.

Nevertheless, before getting to the heart of the matter how to perform a routine reflexology session, we must first discuss the principles behind the methods. Here is an overview of what reflexology is:

Reflexology is supported by a belief system that is different from Western medicine

There is a whole belief system behind the practice. When you're with a professional reflexologist, he or she will tell you that these methods should not be used to replace conventional medicine. It works differently than Western medicine. Instead of replacing one with another, the best practice is to use both when trying to treat an ailment.

You should learn the Eastern principles of life force to be able to practice reflexology effectively. By learning these principles, you will know the benefits and limitations of this healing art.

Reflexology should be practiced even when we are healthy

Unlike Western medicine, reflexology should be practiced even when you are healthy. The principles that reflexology respects promote great health in both body and mind. When practiced consistently, it can prevent disease for years and improve a person's health.

The concepts that govern reflexology were widely accepted in the most ancient civilizations.

It is known that reflexology originated in China. Reflexology tools were among the artifacts found in excavated Chinese tombs. However, the ancient Chinese were not the only group of people who believed in energy flow within the body. The same concepts were believed in ancient Egypt. The same practices of healing pressure were also practiced in this ancient civilization, as suggested in medical scriptures.

Almost all ancient civilizations had their own words referring to the life force. In Chinese, this is referred to as Chi. In Japan, they call this energy Qi. In India, Prana is called.

Modern reflexology makes use of knowledge gained from the past

Modern reflexology is a refined form of the ancient healing ways from Asia. Variations of the method we know today were practiced in ancient civilizations.

Ancient Chinese civilization is the source of the principles of reflexology. Although the idea of a flowing life force within the body is widespread, the Chinese had the most thorough understanding of how it worked and how it can be manipulated for our health.

They believed that life energy flows through our bodies. A disorder or disease begins with an imbalance in this energy flow. For the ancient Chinese, reflexology is as much spiritual as it is medicinal. We only feel it when there is an imbalance, and we need to correct this imbalance or become a disease. Although we cannot observe this form of energy with our current technology, we can use the past knowledge to try to manipulate it for our well-being.

REFLEXOLOGY AIMS TO CREATE BALANCE WITHIN THE BODY

It had been introduced to the West in the early part

of the 20th century. Although Western medicine considers it an alternative form of healing, millions of people have come to believe in its effectiveness.

Most people see reflexology as a form of massage that helps relieve various types of tension. However, it is much more than that. A reflexologist aims to heal various parts of the body by applying pressure to specific points upon the soles of the feet, the palms of the hands, and certain parts of the head. In this way, the reflexologist aims to balance the body's energy flow.

IT IS GENTLE AND USES ONLY TOUCH AND PRESSURE

It is a form of therapy that uses touch and pressure to alleviate certain health conditions. It does not use any form of drugs or even Eastern medicinal herbs. Its main goal is to heal the body, but it also improves circulation, relieves stress, and improves the body's homeostasis.

It also aims to keep the energy flow of certain organs balanced. An experienced reflexologist can access a specific organ by applying pressure to the correct reflex areas.

REFLEXOLOGY CAN BE APPLIED TO ANYONE

Many people think of reflexology as a form of massage. Because of this, they think it is not ideal for pregnant women and children. This is a common misconception. Reflexology can be done to anyone. It aims to make the body more relaxed. If the reflexologist is successful, this can also cause relief for pregnant women.

Reflexology is also allowed in children as their hands and feet become more developed. You should be careful about the degree of pressure you apply because their bones are still soft and developing. The only reason most reflexologists don't apply their techniques to children is that there are better forms of touch therapies that suit the needs of children.

OUR BODY IS AN ENERGY SYSTEMS

Western medicine has not fully embraced reflexology due to the lack of published research to prove its effectiveness. In Western medicine, the body is considered a machine with multiple moving parts. When one part of the machine malfunctions or breaks down, the entire machine fails.

Eastern energy medicine does not refute this; however, its followers also believe that aside from what we can observe by studying anatomy, an invisible force allows our bodies to function perfectly. This force has many names in many cultures. Some refer to it as the life force. In reflexology, this life force is referred to as "Qi."

Eastern energy medicine sees the body as a system

of flowing energy. The flow of Qi is important in keeping the body healthy and functional. When there is a disturbance in our Qi, we feel it immediately. It manifests itself through pain, confusion, and other types of discomfort. Some people prefer to ignore their discomfort and negative feelings. For reflexologists, prolonged imbalance in the flow of Qi is a major contributor to worsening disease and pain.

CHAPTER 2. Qi: What Is It? How It Works?

Qi flow is at the core of reflexology. Many people ignore reflexology as a legitimate healing practice because they fail to grasp what Qi is. In modern times, we define Qi as a life force or energy. This is a simplified definition of the concept for Westerners. Early practitioners of reflexology translated it this way to make it easier to understand in the West.

In Chinese medicine, Qi is a much more complicated concept. In Chinese medical scriptures, Qi is also referred to as a substance at the microscopic level that interacts with molecules in living organisms. Qi is said to be responsible for organizing molecules into organs. The flow of Qi gives life to flesh and blood.

QI IS PRESENT ALL AROUND US

One of the most common questions about Qi is its origins. People want to know where it comes from and how we can get it. Qi is present throughout the universe, and there is never a shortage of it in your environment. It is in all the objects around you in varying amounts. It is in the tree outside your window and in the food you eat.

All of these things have Qi. Qi, however, only flows freely in living organisms. Each person has Qi flowing within his or her body just like blood. You were born with Qi that came from your mother and father. Your body accumulated Qi as you grew up.

We spend Qi every day when we select our daily activities. However, we also replenish it in different ways.

HOW TO REPLENISH QI?

Through the things, we put into our bodies

The science of nutrition has taught us that our bodies need nourishment to function properly. We eat and drink to get the natural resources the body requires to function properly. We also eat to replenish our energy source. The best sources of food for humans are those that come from other living organisms. This is because only these organisms have the Qi we need to continue to function properly.

The quality of food that we put in our body also affects the amount of Qi we receive. The most Qi balanced types of food for us are those that come from plants. The life energy in plants is just enough for our daily needs. Meat is also a good source of Qi.

Across the Universe

As stated earlier in the chapter, Qi is everywhere around us. It is present everywhere in the Universe. You can take the life force from the Universe and make it your own. Some of the techniques allow you to tap into the energy source of the Universe. Some claim that meditation is one of the most effective ways to get Qi from the Universe. There are many forms of meditation. Some religions meditate through repetitive chanting. Others prefer to meditate in silence. You can also get Qi from the Universe by using the meditative practices you have in your religion.

Through the things we do

We can also develop Qi from within our bodies. Practices like yoga and Tai Chi are just two wellness activities designed to develop Qi within the human body.

Other forms of exercise also allow our bodies to create their Qi. Jogging, for example, relaxes our minds.

Along with physical activity, this relaxed state of mind makes conditions conducive to Qi creation. By living an active lifestyle, we give our bodies another source of Qi besides the food we eat, and we get it from the Universe.

WHY DO WE NEED QI?

In Chinese medicine, the difference between dead cells and living cells is the presence of Qi. When certain parts of a living organism lose Qi, they begin to malfunction. When it is depleted, the life form dies, and living matter begins to decay.

From a wellness perspective, Qi flows through our organs to keep them functioning properly. When an organ or portion of the body is not functioning properly, there may be a deficiency or overabundance of Qi in that area.

HOW IS QI RELATED TO REFLEXOLOGY?

When a reflexologist applies pressure to a part of your foot, they try to stimulate the flow of Qi in a specific part of your body. The Chinese have documented the flow of Qi in our bodies. The channels through which Qi flows are called meridians in the Western form of acupuncture. These meridians allow Qi to flow to all parts of your body. These are also the channels touched by acupuncturists when they attach needles to a patient.

In reflexology, we focus on the feet because this is

the area where most of the meridians end. There are also meridian terminations in the palms of our hands and our heads. Some ancient Chinese scriptures suggest that our Qi is connected to the Qi of the earth when our feet touch the ground.

Aside from that, an imbalance in the flow of Qi also affects the body's ability to defend itself, giving way to the onset of disease and infection. Long-term Qi imbalance can lead to a lack of energy and unwillingness to deal with life's complexities.

HOW DOES REFLEXOLOGY HEAL A PERSON?

The role of the reflexologist is to identify areas where there may be a disruption of Qi and to use reflexology to restore the flow of energy. In Chinese energy medicine, harmony in energy flow is the goal. Good health is a sign that the flow of Qi in the body is not blocked.

A reflexologist's role in healing a person is to release their trapped Qi in the area of concern. The reflexologist can do this by adding pressure to the right areas of the palms or soles that are connected to the stomach. He can also apply pressure to the reflex areas of the organs surrounding the organ of concern because there may also be an interruption in the flow of Qi in these areas.

WHAT CAUSES THE INTERRUPTION IN QI FLOW?

There are multiple causes why the flow of energy in our body changes and becomes unbalanced. It can happen due to external factors that affect our health. During these events, the flow of Qi is interrupted. Because it is not flowing freely, some parts of the body may deplete Qi while others may have an excess supply. This imbalance in Qi flow causes the signs and symptoms we feel. These are some of the conditions that cause the energy flux to be interrupted:

1. *Extreme Emotions*

Extreme emotions can also disrupt our Qi flow. Too many negative emotions can lead to disrupted Qi flow in the brain and heart. For example, when we hear bad news, we feel inexplicably stressed. The feeling of stress can be so sudden that we wonder how our mood can change so quickly.

Eastern medicine suggests that a blockage of Qi causes this feeling of stress to our heart or mind. The reflexologist will then attempt to restore balance in these parts by applying pressure to the respective reflex zones. This will bring the fast heart rate back to normal and relax the brain. Skilled reflexologists can also make the mind more relaxed, preventing strong impacts that can result from extreme emotions.

Since this aspect is the most overlooked in conventional forms of medicine, we will discuss it in detail in the next chapter.

1. *Presence of harmful organisms in the body*

Let's take a parasitic infection in the intestines as an example. When a parasite enters our body and multiplies our digestive system, we become weak because we no longer get enough nutrients. This is the explanation of Western medicine. Aside from that, the presence of the parasite also disrupts our energy flow. The microorganisms in our digestive system weaken our Qi along with our nutrition. This causes a systemic decrease in our energy.

1. *Lack of rest*

Parts of our bodies can also experience low Qi levels when we overuse them without giving them time to rest. For example, if you work all night in front of a computer, you may feel the effects of Qi imbalance in your eyes and surrounding body parts. You may also feel discomfort in the brain that controls and manages the sense of sight.

1. *Excessive indulgence in food and other substances*

It can also be caused by overindulgence in the use of certain substances. There would be a disruption in the flow of Qi when we eat too many unhealthy foods. It can also happen when we indulge in too many addictive substances. In the time of the ancient Chinese, opium and alcohol caused most of the damage. Today, hundreds of different natural and artificial substances can cause the flow of Qi to be disrupted.

Chapter Two
CHAPTER 3. BENEFITS

Some of the benefits of reflexology include increasing energy, stimulating nerve function, increasing circulation, eliminating toxins, stimulating the central nervous system, cleansing urinary tract conditions, preventing migraines, relieving pain, reducing depression, relieving sleep disturbances, speeding up recovery after surgery or injury, and inducing a state of deep relaxation. Reflexology can also help make the process of treating certain types of cancer easier. It also soothes the aches and pains of pregnancy, even the aches and pains after the baby are born.

Many people stand all day while working. Whether you work in a field, a factory, an office, a hospital, or any other workplace, there is a chance that you put on stress and weight on your feet daily. Stress can manifest in other parts of the body as well.

The same can be said for back pain. When it comes to the back, people go to the therapist and get a massage, therefore it makes sense that there is one corresponding massage for the foot. Reflexology can be a foot massage, but there is more to it than that. As a specific form of massage therapy, reflexology also includes the ears and hands, making the practice an extremity massage instead of just a foot massage.

While reflexology is primarily used to relieve stress, reflexology can help other areas of the body function optimally.

Energy Levels. By aligning the function of various muscle and organ systems, reflexology can increase energy generation and metabolic processes within the body. If you're sluggish and need a boost of energy, a session can help you gain more energy to do what's necessary. Nerve function. As your body ages, its nerve endings become less sensitive in certain parts, especially in the extremities. Reflexology has been linked to stimulating over 8,000 nerve endings in one session; therefore, increasing nerve responsiveness and function.

Cleaning and opening neural pathways can help improve flexibility and function in many areas of the body. Neural pathways are similar to muscles, and it's always a good idea to give them a workout (via reflexology) from time to time to keep them in great condition.

Relaxation. Reflexology can open neural pathways, and the result of the free-flowing neural act is a more relaxed state of the body, with reduced stress levels. It can make you relaxed by inducing calm in your mind and throughout your body. It can also help treat sleep problems like insomnia, which can be troubling for people who want to get enough rest.

It helps your body relax into a relaxed state and return to its healthy, regular circadian cycles.

Circulation. A verified benefit of the reflexology is for the overall circulation of the body. This means that oxygen and blood are run through the body more efficiently. More oxygen can get to vital organs; therefore, optimizing organ function. In turn, the metabolism is increased. Optimal circulation - with the help of reflexology - also means faster regrowth and healing of damaged cells.

Nervous System Stimulation. Open neural pathways can help the central nervous system in many ways. With reflexology, the brain can effectively handle input, which means the cognitive function will accelerate. It also means that memory will be enhanced, and physical reactions will be smoother and faster. The brain will generally simply work faster and better.

Toxin Removal. Reflexology can alleviate urinary tract problems and improve bladder function. Reflexology can help expel toxins and other foreign substances and protect the body from various health conditions and diseases resulting from an improperly functioning urinary system.

Accelerate healing. The mix of increased circulation and nerve activity and the balanced functioning of metabolism means that cells can regenerate faster and wounds can heal better. The pain-relieving attributes of reflexology can make patients feel better in no time. They are also willing to begin physical recovery to return to the world.

Headaches and Migraines. A lot of people use reflexology as an instrument for eliminating pain. Reflexology, as an analgesic treatment, can reduce headaches and the severity of migraines. This is done simply by relieving muscle tension, which often causes such conditions. Stress-induced headaches can also be eliminated, as psychological factors and stress often manifest in the physical symptoms of migraine.

Before you reach for that Tylenol, you might want to try a reflexology session for your headache. You can also be relaxed afterward.

Menstruation and pregnancy. Research has shown that reflexology can help pregnant women, particularly when it comes to the length of labor and women's needs for pain medication during the postpartum recovery time. It can help reduce a new mother's likelihood of developing postpartum depression. It can also help a woman's body heal faster to resume her regular metabolic activity quickly.

Cancer relief. While reflexology is not a cure for cancer, it can help relieve the side effects of cancer treatments (chemotherapy). It allows patients to reduce anxiety and sleep better. It also reduces indigestion and vomiting problems associated with cancer treatment procedures.

The more general effects of reflexology, such as increasing circulation and clearing neural pathways, may slow the spread of cancer cells and stimulate antioxidants that help destroy cancer cells. However, research continues in this area.

While much of the research on reflexology has not been widely accepted, the reports of success and thousands of traditional uses cannot be ignored. More and more people are still turning to reflexology as an alternative treatment. As such, reflexology should be treated more as a supplemental therapy to medical conditions.

Reflexology is safe, and there is nothing wrong with

using it in conjunction with more conventional treatment of the condition. Just remember to get a qualified reflexologist to help you. Over time, you may be able to use some self reflexology techniques that you may find convenient.

Chapter Three

CHAPTER 4. EXTREME EMOTIONS: THE EFFECTS

In psychology, doctors believe that psychological disorders come from the imbalance of chemicals in the brain. Medications are then used to correct the levels of these chemicals. When balance is achieved, the person can function properly again.

Eastern medicine recognizes the importance of maintaining proper levels of chemicals. However, reflexologists argue that the chemical imbalance in the brain is caused by strong, uncontrolled emotions that have disrupted the person's qi flow in mind. Since there is a disturbance in the flow of qi, the brain and its parts do not function properly in producing these chemicals.

Unless the flow of qi in the brain is fixed, the brain will always need medication to keep these chemicals balanced. This is why reflexologists emphasize the use of this healing process in conjunction with Western medicine. While Western medicine deals with the signs and symptoms, reflexology deals with the underlying causes of long-term healing.

Emotions are not always bad for your Qi flow. It depends on the type of emotion you focus on. Some types of emotions stimulate the balanced flow of Qi. On the other hand, some types of emotions can interrupt it.

Addressing the core of problems

Traditional Eastern medicine states that the cause of emotions is the spirit. We feel what our spirit wants. When the things we do and the things happening around us are not in line with what our spirit wants, we experience negative emotions. Negative emotions in themselves are normal and do not have a lasting effect on the flow of Qi. But if you are in a model of too many negative emotions, this is when your qi flow starts to become unbalanced. If you correct it in time, there will be no negative effects on your body. Disorders will begin to happen when the imbalance is prolonged.

Signs that your emotions are disrupting qi flow

Most people do not know that their extreme emotions are causing their health problems until it is too late. To know if your emotions are causing your qi flow to be unbalanced, you need to observe your reactions towards everyday events. People whose emotions are disrupting their Qi flow tend to over-indulge in negative emotion.

For example, a grieving person is likely to over-indulge in sadness. An irritable person, on the other hand, is likely to over-indulge in anger. Most people are also tempted to let these emotions run free most of the time. However, after a mental wrestling match with the rational side of our brain, we can control these emotions. The people who let these emotions win regularly are the ones whose qi flow is disrupted.

Eastern medicine also relates specific emotions to an organ in the body. For example, the heart is the place of the spirit and is the center of joy. Anger emotion is linked with liver function. The lungs are for anxiety, while the kidney is for fear.

When a person has a problem controlling one of these emotions, its organ may malfunction. The malfunction is caused by the interruption of Qi in this area. When the flow of Qi is not treated, the malfunctioning organ can cause a disorder and even affect the other organs around it.

The role of reflexology in relieving stress

Reflexology can help relieve stress caused by the excess of a certain emotion. For example, we can reduce the effects of anger simply by touching the reflex area of the liver. By pressing on the reflex areas of the lungs, we may be able to reduce a person's anxiety.

This is why we need to make reflexology a habit. By going to a reflexologist regularly, we can also improve our temperament and reduce the stress levels we experience. When we keep all of our emotions controlled, our Qi flow will not be disturbed, and our organs will remain healthy.

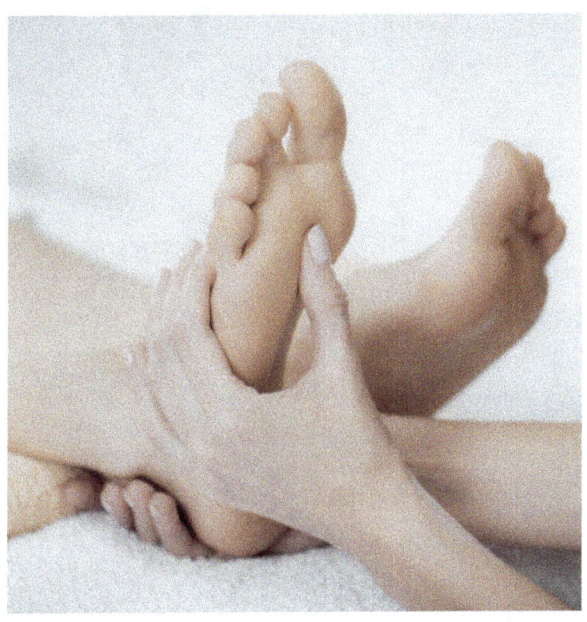

Chapter Four

CHAPTER 5. THE REFLEXOLOGY CHART MAP

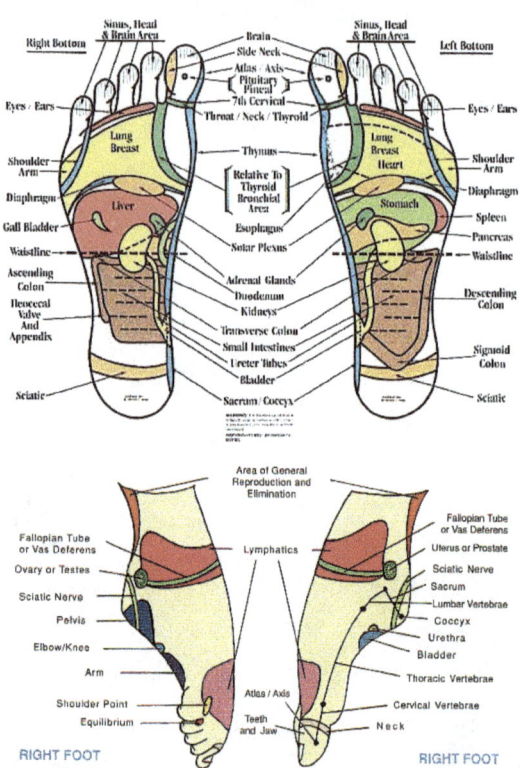

*B*efore starting with reflexology, it is best to know what other alternative therapies are related to it. Some of them are acupressure and acupuncture. Reflexology is similar to both treatments because it influences the vital energy of the human body by stimulating certain points on the body. Acupressure/acupuncture points, however, do not often coincide with the points used by reflexology.

Acupressure and reflexology are both considered "reflex" therapies in that they work with pressure points on one part of the body to affect the other parts of the human body. While reflexology uses reflexes in an orderly fashion that resembles the shape of a human body on the outer ears, hands, and feet, acupressure uses more than 700 reflex points found along the meridians (subtle energy lines) that run the entire length of the body.

Massage is another practice related to reflexology. However, both therapies are sometimes interchanged. While both reflexology and massage use touch, their approaches are not the same.

- Reflexology uses reflex maps of areas and points of the body in the ears, hands, and feet using micro-movement methods such as walking with the fingers or thumb and backing up and looking to generate a response throughout the body.

Massage is the basic manipulation of the body's soft tissues, using special techniques such as friction, stroking, kneading, and tapping to relax the muscles.

Therefore, massage therapists work from the outside to manipulate particular muscle groups to relieve tension. On the other hand, reflexology practitioners work "inside out" to stimulate the central nervous system and release stress.

To practice reflexology effectively, therapists must fully know reflexology maps, which depict the feet (the most commonly used map), hands, and ears. Therapists access these points on the hands and feet (top, sides, and bottom) and at the ear (both outside and inside as far as can be reached) to affect systems and organs throughout the body.

Reflexology maps have been passed among practitioners around the world. There is no agreement on the points among reflexologists. However, there is general agreement on the major reflex points. There is also scientific documentation of the connections between the internal organs and the skin.

To represent how the human body systems correspond to each other, reflexologists use "reflexology charts." Perhaps the most commonly used reflexology chart is for the feet. Each foot is representative of a vertical half of the human body.

- The *right foot* corresponds to the right side of the body and the organs on that side. The liver, for example, is located on the right side of the body, so its designated reflex point is on the right foot.

- The *left foot* is connected to the left side of the body and all the valves and organs on that side.

A reflexologist may do a general integrated session or focus on a particular problem area on the ears, hands, or feet. If there is no time and the person just wants to relax, the therapist can simply work on the ears. Whatever the techniques, reflexologists believe they are releasing stress or congestion in the nervous system, thus balancing the body's energy.

REFLEX ZONES IN THE FEET
The Toes

The brain is located in the upper part of the body. It occupies both the right and left sides of the head. Your reflex zone is also located on the tips of your toes. When you feel you have a qi imbalance in your head, you should apply pressure to the tips of your toes and other toes.

All other parts of the head have their reflex points in the toes. The nose has a left side and a right side. Their reflex zones are located on the outer side of the all. It is near the reflex zone of the brain, which is located on the tip of the finger. The glands surrounding the nose are also located in the middle of the allium.

The eyes also have a left and right side. Their reflex zones are located in the middle of the two fingers next to the big toe. If you feel that your eyes have a qi imbalance, you should apply pressure to the skin under these two fingers in each foot. The same sections of the last two fingers are the reflex zones for the sinuses. The reflex zone of the throat is located in the allium joint. The reflex zones of the neck, in general, are located in the joints of the smaller toes.

The ball of the soles also has many reflex zones for the organs just below the head. Directly behind the small toe is the reflex area of the arms and shoulders. The reflex areas of each lung are located behind the joints of the three middle fingers. There is a line connecting the pupil joint to the outer side of the foot. This line is the reflex zone for our bronchial organs. The reflex zone of the heart is located in the ball of the foot directly behind the toe.

The Arch of the Soles

The reflex zones of the organs in our abdominal area are located in the middle of the soles. Just behind the reflex zones of the lungs is the zone for the diaphragm. It is thinner than the other reflex zones.

The soft area of the sole is the reflex zone for most of

our organs related to digestion. In the left foot, the complete middle part is dominated by the gallbladder reflex area. The same area of the right foot is shared by the reflex zones of the spleen, stomach, liver, and pancreas. The outermost side is for the spleen. The center of the soft area is the stomach and pancreas. The innermost side is for the liver. The center of the soft area in both feet is for the two kidneys. The inner side of the left sole in the area for the adrenal glands.

The areas between the soft part of the sole and the heel are the reflex zones for the gut. The area for the colon surrounds this area, while the center is the area for the small intestine.

The Heel

The heel contains fewer reflex zones. You should apply pressure in a line across the heels to improve the flow of qi into the sciatic nerves. Just behind this line is the reflex area of the left and right pelvis. Just above the sciatic nerve area in the left foot is the area for the appendix.

To locate the reflex zones more accurately, you can trace your feet on paper and use a reflex zone diagram. Use the reflex zone diagram to identify the different areas of your foot. Draw different zones in the contour of your foot on the piece of paper.

Hand Reflexology

The palms of the hands may be as well used for reflexology. Just as in the foot, reflex zones for the head, brain, and sinuses can be located in the fingertips. The tips of the thumbs are specific to the pituitary gland. The middle of the fingers is for the neck and throat area, while the joints of all fingers are for the eyes and ears.

The parts of the palms just below the knuckles are for your two lungs. In the left hand, the heart shares the area for the lung. The center of the palms on the left hand is for the stomach. On the right hand, the same area is for the liver. The colon and small intestine share the parts closest to the wrist. For a more detailed study of the reflex zones in your hands, you should also trace the outline of your hands on a piece of paper and create a cheat sheet by drawing the reflex zones in it.

How to apply pressure?

When using reflexology in the hands or feet, the goal is to locate the reflex area you need to apply pressure. You should then use your thumb to locate knots that may have formed in this area due to Qi buildup. This technique is referred to as a thumb walk. You do this by lightly pressing the reflex areas with your thumb, letting it glide across the area. You should press lightly to feel what is under the skin.

At first, you might find it tough locate these nodes. To teach yourself to find them, you should press the same areas on each foot. You may feel a difference between the two areas. You can also ask the person as you are pressing if they feel a difference in the pressure you apply.

When locating knots in the reflex area, the goal is to massage this area with your thumb. Knots tend to break down with continued pressure on the area. If the skin on your thumbs is too soft, you may not be able to apply enough pressure to affect the knots in the reflex zones. In this case, you can use tools to apply pressure.

In the past, Chinese doctors used smooth stone or wooden instruments that resembled the shape of the thumb. These days, there are many wooden and rubber reflexology instruments on the market. They come in various shapes and sizes. All, however, have a protrusion that simulates the thumb. This end is pushed toward the skin to create pressure.

Whether using your thumb or a reflexology tool, you should learn how to apply pressure to the specific area properly. Be sure to apply enough pressure without causing the person pain. If the person is in pain with the pressure, it will cause some distress in him and may interrupt his qi flow.

You need to find the right amount of pressure. When performing a reflexology session with someone, you need to communicate with them to know their pressure threshold at the beginning of the session.

When you have found the right amount of pressure, your goal is to apply it to the reflex areas where you find the nodes. You should apply pressure in a circular motion in these nodes. You should first practice this circular motion on your feet to be able to improve your skills.

The right environment for reflexology

When you are doing reflexology techniques to yourself, you should prepare the right environment and relax.

Choose a room without bright colors. Bright colors like bright red, orange and yellow are straining your eyes. You should also avoid an overly bright room with white walls. Whenever possible, opt for a room with plenty of natural light and walls with earthy colors.

The temperature should be just right. The seat should also be as comfortable as possible.

There should not be a strong odor in the air. If you're masking a strong smell, be sure to use scents that simulate the smell of nature to make it more relaxing.

As far as sound goes, silence is best. However, if you can't achieve this, you can mask other sounds with nature's white noise. Or you can ask who you are treating for the music or sound that makes them more relaxed.

In the end, you should work with what you have and be sure to remove anything that might distract a person from relaxation. There should be no access to distracting electronic devices such as cell phones or tablets throughout reflexology sessions. The strong glow from these types of devices is too strong for the eyes. It can cause distress.

Frequency of Reflexology

Reflexology can be done every day if you have time. Doing it once a day will keep your Qi flow balanced throughout the week.

Chapter Five

CHAPTER 6. HOW TO PRACTICE REFLEXOLOGY

If you want to try reflexology to relax or pair it with any existing therapy you might use, you should know what happens in a typical reflexology session. You should also know what its guiding principles are.

The body responds to touch, which can help facilitate healing on multiple levels. Reflexology clients can often think they need to "focus" or "concentrate" to feel the benefits of the practice. While calmness will induce deeper feelings, you don't need to have special habits or skills for reflexology to be effective. As long as the reflexologist knows what he or she is doing, allows the energy to flow, and stays centered, you - the client - can respond positively.

The body heals itself; reflexologists only help to

promote the healing process. Instead of being the "healer," the reflexologist is just a participant in the reflexology session. Practitioners need to ground and center themselves and thus allow the client to "heal" themselves.

This recognition that reflexology is meant to help balance the person so that the human body can repair and nourish itself. A practitioner recognizes that the purpose of reflexology is to help the client align their energy and self-healing ability.

Clients and practitioners can feel the movement of energy. A reflexology practitioner can feel the flow of energy from a pressure point on the hands, ears, or feet to the rest of the body. When working on the gallbladder and spleen points, for example, the reflexologist can feel a flow of energy and access the points simultaneously. Because of the power of the two points, the client can also feel the flow of energy.

Human beings are made up of an emotional and physical body, with a spirit and mind interdependent. The reflexologist considers all aspects of the client's being: spirit, mind, emotion, and body. A relaxed body can induce a calm mind, an integrated spirit, and calm emotions.

Now that you know what the principles of reflexology are learn more about what happens in a reflexology session. A typical session begins with the practitioner taking a health history to determine if reflexology is the best course of therapeutic action.

The practitioner explains to you how the practice works and what happens during a reflexology session. They also inform you that the practice is not a substitute for medical treatment and does not treat a particular disease. Some practitioners may ask you to sign a waiver or consent form. After doing so, the session begins.

Depending on your particular health problem, the reflexologist may choose to work only on your hands, ears, or feet. There are also some situations where a patient confined to a hospital may get a food reflex session, even if he/she is attached to multiple IV tubes and other wires and tubes.

It is best if the reflexologist decides what type of therapy will be worked on you. If the therapist chooses to work on your feet, you will sit or lie down and be fully dressed, except for socks and footwear. The reflexologist will wash and soak your feet in warm water, then place them at your chest level.

The practitioner will begin by checking your feet for sores, rashes, open wounds, bursitis, or plantar warts and will ask about any leg or foot pain that may be hindering the therapy. As mentioned earlier, a reflexology session lasts anywhere from 30 minutes to an hour. At your discretion, you can talk or rest during the session. You will still get the benefits of the treatment even if you fall asleep during the therapy session.

While the session is in progress, feedback is encouraged, and you can even request to stop the reflexology session at any time if you experience pain.

The Reflexology Treatment

A full therapy session uses various techniques and includes points on both feet (perhaps ears and hands as well). The reflexology session begins at the toes or fingers and works toward the heel of the foot or hand, then works the top and sides of the area being worked on.

As the reflexologist works on the pressure points, he or she targets the glands and internal organs and the bones, muscle groups, nerve ganglia (brachial plexus, solar plexus), and sciatic nerves during the session. If tension or congestion is found during a session, the reflexologist will apply pressure to balance the body.

If there is an area of pain, that area is worked on until that point or area reaches harmony. Release of pain is not the goal. Instead, it brings the human body into balance so that the pain will disappear. The nervous system will be stimulated to do the work. When the session ends, the therapist can then return to that point or area to confirm whether or not the pain has disappeared.

Ending the session

Many reflexologists have a peaceful and calm way to end the session that involves stroking the foot or hand and holding that limb in a particular way. It is important to feel nurtured and comforted. It is also important to have felt relaxed during the session.

You should not feel rushed or start rushing to do things once the session is over—Orient yourself by gently returning to the present. While you are in a comfortable state, gather yourself slowly to leave the place refreshed. We recommend drinking water and being aware of your body over the next few hours. If you have any questions or concerns, please feel free to raise them to your practitioner.

During a session, you may experience some reactions. Many of the reactions are good signs that the therapy is working. Some of the symptoms that normally last for a day or two indicate the human body's attempt to return to a state of harmony and balance. Some of the reactions may include:

- Improved sleep
- Increased energy
- More mobile joints
- Pain

- Fatigue
- Kidney stones are passed effortlessly
- Pimples, spots, or rashes (due to the elimination of toxins)
- Increased mucus (vaginal or nasal discharge)
- Diarrhea, frequent bowel movements (toxin elimination, cleansing)
- Psychological or emotional release (crying)
- Flu-like symptoms

Required Sessions

The number of reflexology sessions needed varies and is usually determined by the client's reasons for seeking reflexology and health. Generally, the results of reflexology sessions are cumulative and subtle, so it would be best to seek multiple sessions, such as once a week for two months.

If you have a specific condition or disease, you may need more sessions. The usual recommendation may be to start with one session each week for six to eight weeks. After that, follow with one session for each month.

Not a diagnosis

Many people may mistake a reflexology session for a diagnosis of a specific disease. No, it isn't. During a reflexology session, reflexologists do not inform you of any tension or congestion they might discover on your hand, ear, or foot that might indicate abnormalities.

A reflexology theory is that the human body will repair and nourish itself once the stress is released. If your body is overstressed, you may be referred to another treatment or medical team when appropriate. A reflexologist cannot diagnose an illness or hand out medical advice.

Chapter Six

CHAPTER 7. THE WHOLE-BODY REFLEXOLOGY

As a beginner, you should not take responsibility for curing a person of serious illness. Your goal is to heal his spirit and the flow of his qi. If he has urgent health problems, you should lead him to health professionals.

Identify the parts of the body that need the most attention

After building rapport and interviewing the person, you should identify the organs you need to give the most attention to. If the person is upset all the time, for example, you should focus on the reflex area of the liver to prevent that emotion from getting out of control.

Prepare what you need

When doing reflexology on yourself or another

person, you should first prepare them physically and mentally. Your goal during preparation is to keep the session hygienic and to make the person feel comfortable. You should also prepare your tools so that they are within your reach right when you need them.

Here's a process you can follow to prepare for a reflexology session.

1. Wash your feet and examine them for wounds

If there are calloused areas, a foot scrub can remove excess skin. The skin on the soles absorbs water quite well and becomes softer immediately after washing. This will make the area more sensitive to pressure.

After washing, you should also check the foot for wounds or other forms of injury. Ask the person if there are any areas you should avoid. Some injuries are not visible on the outside.

1. Lengthen the spine

Let the patient stretch their back by standing up straight and extending their arms upward until they are at the tips of their toes. If done correctly, this will lengthen the spine, allowing better circulation of qi.

1. Instruct the patient to do a deep breathing exercise.

Tell him or her to take three deep breaths and ten normal breaths. When breathing normally, instruct the person to try to relax the mind. He needs to remove all thoughts that might be bothering him. If he cannot empty his mind, tell him to count his breaths from one to ten.

1. Loosen the joints in each foot

Roll up each foot to loosen the joints. Extend the heels by pushing the ball of the foot toward the patient's body. Make the opposite motion by pulling on the foot.

If you are prepping your foot, you can use a flat rubber band or piece of towel to stretch the heels. Place the middle of the towel into the ball of your foot while holding each end with your hands. You should then lean back as you pull the ends of the towel to bend your foot closer to your body.

You can also stretch this area by using the steps of the stairs. On the edge of the bottom step of the stairs, stand on the ball of one foot. You should then allow gravity to pull your heels closer to the ground as the ball of your foot supports your full weight. If done correctly, you will feel the heels and plantar area of the foot stretch.

1. Let the person relax

Finally, you should let the person sit and relax. The legs should be extended toward you. The arms should also be extended with the palms wide open. You should also instruct the person to breathe with their stomach while they are relaxing.

When all of this is done, you should begin with the session. Here is a process you can follow:

1. Start with the toes and work your way down to the heel.

The best way to start is to do a thumb walk of all the reflex zones in one foot. You should use both thumbs to apply gentle pressure on the person's sole. Start with the tips of the fingers or toes. This is the area for the head. As you move lower, you are scanning the entire body from head to fingers with your thumbs.

Your first goal when doing this is to assess the hardness of the skin and the right amount of pressure to apply. You should ask the person if the pressure is too weak or too strong. You can then adjust the strength of the pressure accordingly.

Your second goal is to scan the reflex areas of the organs of interest. You should already be looking for areas where the flesh is stiff. If the sole is too calloused for you, you can wipe the foot with a warm cloth. This will make the skin temporarily softer.

1. Locate the reflex zones of the organs you are concerned with

After walking your thumb through your entire foot, you should return to the reflex zones of the problem organs. If you are not familiar with the location of the reflex zone, then you should have a map of the reflex zones at your side. You should then walk with your thumb in this area. Your goal is to find the stiffest part of the area and apply pressure to it. In addition to gently pressing this area, you should also try to apply a circular motion on it.

You should start with weaker pressure on these areas. You can then gradually increase the pressure and ask the person to call your attention if the pressure becomes too painful.

1. Prepare your hands and work on them

After working on your feet, you should prepare your hands as well. You should also walk your thumb from your fingertips to your wrist. Since palms tend to be softer than soles, you need to apply less pressure on them.

1. Identify reflex zones

You should do the same process to your hand. First, you should locate the reflex zone of the organ you need to work on. You then need to apply pressure on these areas to locate the part with the most stiffness. When you have located it, apply pressure to it in a circular motion.

People who do not attend reflexology sessions regularly are more sensitive to the change in Qi flow when they undergo a reflexology session. Those who are used to reflexology, on the other hand, will be less sensitive to your touch. In this case, you may need to apply more pressure to your hands and feet.

During the session, you need to communicate with the person you are providing the service too. Keep them calm and observe their reactions. If they are giving expressions of pain, then you may need to reduce the pressure you apply. If they are not giving any facial reactions, you need to ask them if the pressure is too weak. Ideally, you should not use oils to reduce friction. However, if you think the session will take a long time, you may need them to keep skin temperature from rising and prevent skin inflammation from too much friction.

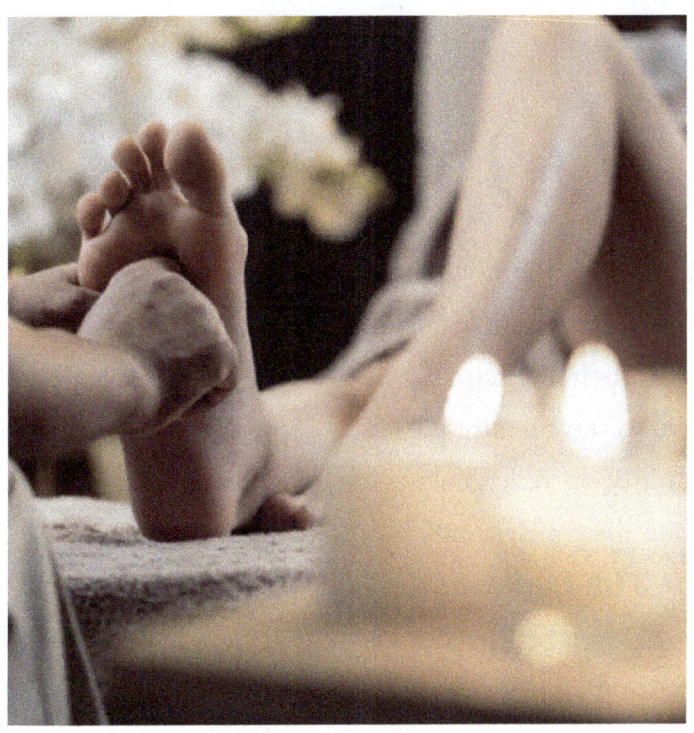

Chapter Seven

CHAPTER 8. REFLEXOLOGY TECHNIQUES

With its ancient origins and rich history, it's no wonder that reflexology is an alternative therapy with a wide range of approaches and methods. The West and the East have each come up with their particular styles of reflexology that are effective. New techniques and approaches are evolving rapidly as reflexologists worldwide develop and share their discoveries and clinical experiences.

The Ingham Method

Developed by Eunice Ingham, a physical therapist, the Ingham Method is the basis for modern reflexology. Mrs. Ingham is considered the "Mother of Reflexology" by many reflexologists. With the Ingham way, pressure is applied by "thumb-walking." In this way, the finger or thumb straightens and bends while maintaining constant pressure on the foot, hand, or ear area being worked on.

Here, the reflexology practitioner uses talcum powder, and a particular session can last for up to an hour, depending on the client's health. The goal of the Ingham method is to balance the body's systems and promote relaxation. The practitioner works within the client's pain tolerance level. In the holistic reflexology session, all reflexes are worked on - some are working on more than others.

The Rwo Shur method

In many areas of Asia, especially in Singapore, China, and Taiwan, the Rwo Shur method of reflexology is implemented. It combines thumb pressure and sliding techniques, incorporates knuckles, and uses small wooden sticks. The therapist applies firm pressure and uses cream, which allows for efficient, smooth, and fast movement.

The session normally lasts half an hour and focuses on stimulation rather than relaxation. In Taiwan, this method was developed by Fr. Joseph Eugster, a Swiss missionary. After experiencing the benefits of reflexology firsthand, Fr. Eugster saw the need to help people with the simple method of reflexology. He then began to treat and teach others this type of reflexology.

Ayurvedic Reflexology

This type of Reflexology, which is based on the principles of Ayurveda, is best described as a successful combination of Western and Eastern techniques and philosophies. Ayurveda is the comprehensive, traditional and ancient medical system of India. Ayurveda-based Reflexology offers practitioners an exciting new approach to working with hands and feet. Sharon Stathis, in Australia, developed the method, which is now routinely used in at least 15 countries.

The approach of Ayurvedic Reflexology is to help balance the body's subtle energy systems by supporting the efficient flow of prana (life energy). Prana flows through the body via the nadis (micro energy channels). In Ayurvedic teachings, the mind and body cannot be healthy if the flow of prana is interrupted or slow.

Located along the nadis are marma points (energy centers) that help maintain the optimal flow of prana. Marma points are located on the vital nadis in each foot and hand. The entire body benefits from working on these points in

Ayurvedic Reflexology sitting hands and feet.

The therapist must use oil when working on the marma points, as unnecessary friction can upset the delicate energy balance. In Ayurvedic Reflexology, warm sesame oil is commonly used. The best type of oil is unbleached, non-deodorized, organic, and cold-pressed. The oil provides the practitioner with the lubrication to work on the marma points. The oil is also the best base for smooth, fast movements attributed to this type of therapy.

Ayurvedic Reflexology can be gentler on the therapist's hands than the traditional "thumb-walking" method of Reflexology. The application, overall, is brisk, but the effect is complete relaxation. During such a session, each foot or hand is fully worked on. An Ayurvedic reflexology session can last from 40 to 45 minutes.

New approaches

In recent years in the West, reflexology practitioners have been looking for ways to balance and influence the body's subtle energies through the hands and feet. Acupressure concepts and points related to energy therapies are increasingly being used in reflexology sessions.

Ancient Chinese teachings are the basis for new approaches where considering principles such as yin/yang, five-phase theory, and meridians is taking holistic treatment to new levels. Special oils, magnets, and colors in a crystal flashlight are sometimes applied to reflex points. Many practitioners will include gentle manipulation that connects the reflexes to balance and encourage the flow of energy.

Although not entirely new, ear and hand reflexology are now widely used in conjunction with foot reflexology. Practitioners can use hand, ear, or foot reflexology in a session. They can also choose the reflex area they feel is right for the client. Reflexologists are now trained in various techniques and methods. This means that a reflexology practitioner can provide you with a session that suits your specific needs.

Chapter Eight
CONCLUSIONS

Reflexology can help restore harmony and balance in the body. It can also release tension. Practitioners believe that reflexology can help facilitate relaxation, a calm mind, and even calmer emotions. Many people describe an unprecedented sense of calm and increased energy after their reflexology sessions. Additionally, specific studies determine that reflexology can reduce anxiety and pain.

Many reflexology users have experienced positive results with their therapy sessions. One cancer patient used reflexology to help him deal with his chemically induced nausea. After undergoing a reflexology session, this user felt more at peace and connected; thus, he was no longer afraid of what he was going through.

The next step is to continue to work on your skills in

applying pressure and locating the reflex zones. At first, you may need to consult your cheat sheet regularly. As you become more proficient, you will be able to locate the reflex zones on your own.

You should also learn to develop the ability to communicate with the person you are treating during the session. This will make them feel comfortable. The effects of reflexology will be greatest when the person is relaxed.

Many people go through reflexology for various reasons. There are also research studies on reflexology being able to help with various medical conditions. There are also ongoing studies on the positive connection of reflexology to medical conditions such as cancer, anxiety, type II diabetes, cardiovascular problems, tension headaches/ migraines, multiple sclerosis, and sinusitis. However, reflexology as a treatment for these conditions is still being solved, and nothing is proven yet.

For now, however, reflexology is an important aid in relieving symptoms. It can be an alternative way to maintain your overall health. Most importantly, reflexology can induce calm and relaxation, and - in today's stressful world - that's what many people need most.

www.ingramcontent.com/pod-product-compliance
Lightning Source LLC
Chambersburg PA
CBHW071125030426
42336CB00013BA/2209